Smart Generation: Technology, Education and the Wellbeing of Youth

Strategies for Managing the Impact of the Internet and Social Media on Youth Development.

introduction

Welcome to the world of "Smart Generation: Youth Technology, Education, and Wellness!" As you well know, this is a world in which smartphones have become our digital appendages, social media is our social stage, and the Internet has become our information universe. In this book, we will explore how the pervasive use of these technologies is shaping the minds and lives of the younger generation, including the impact on very young children.

In recent decades, we have witnessed an incredible acceleration in the growth and adoption of digital technology. Today's youth have grown up in an environment where the digital world is an integral part of their existence.
Smartphones, tablets and laptops have become indispensable tools in daily life, allowing instant access to a wide range of information and social connections.

But with this digital revolution, new questions and challenges have also emerged. How do technology and social media affect the mental health of young people? Is the cognitive development of young children affected? What are the risks and opportunities related to online safety? How is the very concept of relationship and communication changing in the digital age? These are just some of the questions we will try to explore in this book.

Our goal is to provide a comprehensive and balanced overview of the implications of technology on the digital generation, examining both the positive and negative aspects.

We want to help you better understand how to navigate this ever-evolving digital world, offering practical tools and advice to meet the challenges and capitalize on the opportunities that technology offers.

In "Smart Generation," you will not only find a wealth of data and statistics, but also stories and personal experiences that will show you how technology really affects the lives of young people. I hope that this book will provide you with not only a greater awareness of these crucial issues, but also insights to promote healthy and conscious use of technology in the younger generation. Get ready to explore the digital world through the eyes of the "Smart Generation"!

Chapter 1: Evolution of Technology and Youth Habits

The dawn of technology

Let's start with the birth of everything; in the 1940s and 1950s, there was a huge breakthrough in the air-the foundation was being laid for what would become the digital world of today that we all know and exploit. This is when ENIAC made its grand entrance. For those who don't know, the ENIAC (Electronic Numerical Integrator and Computer) was kind of the granddaddy of all modern computers. It was built by a group of brains at the University of Pennsylvania, John Mauchly and J. Presper Eckert.

Now, obviously don't expect anything like your smartphone or laptop. The ENIAC was huge, taking up a space the size of a room and weighing tons - literally! And imagine, we are not talking about one or two pieces, but more than 17,000 thermionic valves! A small city of tubes, so to speak.

His first mission? Calculating the trajectories of bullets during World War II. But once ENIAC made its first moves, there was very little it could not do. It helped launch the era of large-scale electronic computation. You can imagine its impact-it changed the way we do computation, solve complex problems, and even the way we communicate.

Now, it was not all sunshine and roses. ENIAC was like a beast to tame-it required a lot of electricity and could overheat faster than an oven. But with all that, it left its mark. It inspired the creation of a series of other computers, each smarter and smaller than the last.

And ENIAC was not only a stepping stone for technological evolution. It changed the way we see the world. It opened doors to new jobs, new industries, and accelerated scientific research. It practically laid the foundation for everything we use today-from social media to driverless cars.

In short, the ENIAC was the rebellious grandfather of the computer family. A pioneer who paved the way for our digital world. Despite its flaws, it is hard to imagine where we would be today without it.

In the 1960s, however, things were really heating up in the world of technology. It's like everyone was saying, "Hey, we really need to make these computers friendlier and easier to use!" And that's really where Fortran comes in.

Imagine Fortran as the first serious attempt to make programming less complicated. Before it, writing code was like a journey into the unknown, full of obscure and complex languages. But Fortran came like a fresh wind, with a syntax closer to English and a more intuitive structure.
It was like learning a new language, but a language that could make computers do amazing things.

And then there is the advent of microprocessors. These little wonders of silicon revolutionized the world of computers. Before them, computers were big, expensive and secretive mainly to governments and large corporations. But with microprocessors, computers have become smaller, faster and more affordable for everyone.

Imagine having the computing power of an ENIAC, but in a fraction of the size and cost. These tiny silicon chips opened the door to a new era of personal computers. Now, even the average boy or girl could afford a computer and use it to do amazing things-from calculating complex equations to creating digital art.

In essence, the 1960s was a time of revolution in the world of technology. With the introduction of Fortran and microprocessors, computers became more affordable and more powerful than ever before. These developments laid the foundation for the digital world we know today, forever changing the way we live, work and play.

Personal Information Technology Revolution

Then came the 1970s, an era of bell-bottoms, long hair and... garage-made computers! Yes, you heard that right! It was during this decade that the computer revolution really began to take off, thanks to a group of passionate geeks who brought computers directly into the homes of ordinary people.

Meet the Altair 8800-the first true PC. Now, don't expect a sleek, slim design like today's laptops. The Altair looked more like a shoebox with lots of buttons and colored lights. But did you know what? It was our first step into the digital revolution.

And then there is the Apple I. Created in the legendary garage of Steve Jobs and Steve Wozniak, this was the real do-it-yourself of the computer world. It was like the Robin Hood of computers-it brought the power of technology into the hands of ordinary people. Although not yet a superpower at the time, the Apple I laid the foundation for what would become one of the world's largest companies.

Imagine the lightning strike of anyone who saw one of these for the first time. On the one hand, it was like, "What the hell is this?" but on the other, it was like, "Wow, I can do what?!" It was as if a whole galaxy of possibilities had opened up before your eyes.

Basically, the 1970s was the time when computers went from being huge, expensive machines to something you could have in your room. And it all started with the Altair 8800 and the Apple I. These pioneers paved the way for a digital future in which everyone from college kids to professionals, they could have had the power of technology at their fingertips.

The Internet Revolution

Ah, the 1980s, the era of bright colors, electronic music and...
Of the incredible digital revolution! And do you know what was
the stroke of genius of those years? The Transmission Control
Protocol/Internet Protocol (TCP/IP) and the World Wide Web
(WWW)! These two literally opened the door to what we now
call the Internet.

So what does all this TCP/IP protocol mean? Simply put, it's like
the secret language that computers use to communicate with
each other on a network. Imagine that computers speak different
dialects, but TCP/IP is like the translator that makes them
understand each other. Without it, the Internet would be a chaos
of computers that don't know what to do with each other.

And then there is the World Wide Web, the epic invention of
Tim Berners- Lee. Before the WWW, surfing the Internet was
like looking for a needle in a haystack. You had to know
exactly the address of what you wanted to find, otherwise you
were lost. But the WWW has changed all that. It's as if Tim
opened a magic door that took you anywhere on the Web with
a single click.

Suddenly, the Internet was no longer just for academics and
the military. It had become a kind of promised land for anyone
who wanted to explore. You could chat with people on the
other side of the world, watch videos of cats doing strange
things, and even go shopping without ever leaving the couch!

In short, thanks to the TCP/IP protocol and the World Wide
Web, the Internet has taken a leap forward and conquered the
world. And the great thing is that this is just the beginning. Who
would have imagined that those two simple (but very powerful)

developments in the 1980s.

Would they have changed the world so much? The Internet has become a kind of parallel universe, where we can do almost anything on our minds, at the click of a button. And all this, thanks to the 1980s!

We delve into the 1990s, the age of opposites: from colorful and eccentric clothing to grunge music, and from the beginning of globalization to the rise of digital culture. But what really made the difference? Web browsers like Netscape Navigator and Internet Explorer!

Imagine this: you're standing there in your living room with a modem that's "creaking" as it connects, and finally, when it looks like the whole world is about to collapse, along comes Netscape Navigator! It was like the Robin Hood of the Internet - it brought the magic of the Web right into the palm of your hands. With its intuitive design and cutting-edge features, it made surfing the Internet a breeze for everyone from nerds to novices.

But wait, let's not forget good old Internet Explorer! It was like the big brother we all had. You can be sure that if you weren't using Netscape, you were definitely browsing with Internet Explorer. Although at first it was a bit like the least loved child of the browser family, it became more and more popular as time went on, until it became an indispensable part of your Internet browsing experience.

With Netscape Navigator and Internet Explorer, the Internet became more accessible and user-friendly than ever before. You no longer had to be a technological genius to navigate the Web - just a couple of clicks and the world was at your feet. Web sites were like open books, ready to be explored, and you were the captain of your digital ship.

So, thanks to these amazing browsers, the 1990s was the era when the Internet really became a force to be reckoned with. It opened the door to a world of opportunity and knowledge, and forever changed the way we connect and interact with the world around us. What a wonderful time!

Age of Smartphones and Social Media

The 2000s, the decade when technology really took off! And do you know what was the real star of this period? Smartphones! Yes, those very magical little devices that we carry everywhere and have become practically an extension of ourselves.

But let's go back to 2007, the year Apple's iPhone was released. It was as if the whole world held its breath as Steve Jobs walked on stage and unveiled this technological jewel. And what a jewel it was! With its sleek design, revolutionary touchscreen and a whole world of apps at your fingertips, the iPhone changed everything. From that moment on, there was never a time when we didn't have access to the Internet, and not just at home, but everywhere!

And then there were the first Android devices, which turned the competition on its head. With their wide range of models and prices, they brought the power of smartphones into the hands of even more people. From students to professionals, from tech enthusiasts to grandparents, everyone wanted a piece of this technological pie.

Smartphones have transformed our daily lives in ways we could not even have imagined. From simple Internet browsing to social media monitoring (social media? We'll get back to that shortly), from e- mail management to GPS navigation, these little devices have become our digital handymen. And let's not forget the apps! With an app for everything from trip planning to meditation, we had the whole world literally at our fingertips.

But there's more! Smartphones have also changed the way we connect with others. There are no more distances - with a call or a text, we can be in touch with anyone, anywhere in the world. And thanks to the built-in camera, we can capture and share the most precious moments of our lives in an instant.

Ah, the 10s of the new millennium, the decade when social media took over the world! It was like a digital explosion that radically changed the way we connect, communicate and share our lives.

Let's talk about Facebook, the granddaddy of all social media. It was the pioneer that paved the way for our digital addiction. With its profile pages, news feeds, and ability to connect with friends and family around the world, Facebook has become the center of our online lives. Who would have thought that such a simple platform could have such an enormous impact on the way we live?

But Facebook was just the beginning. Then came Twitter and Instagram to revolutionize the game even more. Twitter took our communication to new heights with its short tweets and hashtags, while Instagram turned photo sharing into an art. With filters and hashtags, every moment of our lives could become a digital masterpiece to share with the world.

And let's not forget YouTube, the king of online videos! It has become the place where we can find just about anything, from makeup tutorials to video game reviews to videos of cats doing funny things(i cats rule the Web!). It has been like having a personalized TV that follows us wherever we go.

But as every coin has its downside, social media has also brought with it new challenges .Cyberbullying and the spread of fake news have become more and more prevalent problems, but sotespecially addictions and live social networking.

In fact, kids don't have to wait to see each other to socialize-you'll say: but there was text messaging before! Yes, but at least the rates were prohibitively expensive for teens, which led them to centering each and every message, but with the advent of Internet-connected smartphones, and consequently Whatsapp and the media mentioned above, teens have begun to be perpetually connected! This leads teens to communicate much less in person (you will have already seen many times a group of teens/teens with Smartphones constantly in their hands who do not interject with each other but all stand mute with their heads in the screen), plus there is another possible problem. access to billions of content leads teens to have already seen everything-or almost everything-at a very young age, leading them to easy boredom and overwhelm. In addition, the constant viewing of rich or perfect-bodied influencers can easily lead young boys to the risk of rushing comparisons, resulting in performance anxiety or even lead them to become depressed.

In short, the 2010s were the decade in which social media took over, transforming the way we live, work and communicate. Whether for good or bad, one thing is certain: we can no longer imagine a life without them.

Emerging Technologies

We all thought we had seen the digital revolution, instead it seems to have not yet stopped! We have arrived at the present, the 2020s. the decade in which emerging technologies have taken the stage and peeped into our daily lives in ways we could have only dreamed of before!
We are talking about things like artificial intelligence (AI), virtual reality (VR) and blockchain. These technologies are not only revolutionizing the way we interact with the digital world, but they are also paving the way for new opportunities and challenges for future generations.

Let's start with artificial intelligence (AI). Yes, just like in science fiction movies, AI is increasingly becoming an integral part of our lives. From personal assistants like Siri and Alexa to self-driving cars, AI is changing the way we live, work and play. It is helping to solve complex problems, improve efficiency and even predict the future. But, of course, it also brings with it some important questions about privacy, ethics and the impact on work. In short, AI is one of those technologies that makes us excited and a little afraid at the same time!

Then there is virtual reality (VR). Who would have thought that we could put on a pair of glasses and immerse ourselves in virtual worlds? Thanks to VR, we can have experiences that were previously impossible, such as traveling through space, exploring ancient ruins or even participating in interactive games as if we were there in person. But it's not just for entertainment - VR is finding applications in areas such as education, health mental and vocational training. It is as if we have an open window to a universe of possibilities!

Finally, let's talk about blockchain. This technology is the foundation of Bitcoin and other cryptocurrencies, but it goes far beyond the world of finance. The blockchain is a decentralized digital ledger that records transactions securely and transparently. This means it can be used for everything from tracking supplies to verifying the authenticity of assets. It is revolutionizing industries such as logistics, healthcare and even the arts. But, of course, it also brings with it questions about security, scalability and legal implications.

In short, the 2020s were the decade when emerging technologies took over. We are heading toward a more advanced digital future, but there are also new challenges ahead of us along the way. So, let's get ready for an exciting journey into the world of technology!

Changes in Daily Habits.

let's get to the heart of the matter-how the advent of technology has changed our daily habits, especially among young people. It's as if we've all become addicted to those little glowing screens in our pockets, isn't it?

So let's take smartphones. Remember when we used them only for calling and texting? Well, now they have become like our digital best friend. We use them for everything from waking up in the morning to instant messaging with friends, from searching for information on Google to listening to our favorite streaming music. It's as if we can't imagine life without them!

What about social media? Well, it has become like our favorite pastime. We spend hours scrolling through Instagram feeds, sharing memes on Facebook, and tweeting on Twitter. It has become a way to stay in touch with friends, but also to explore new ideas, trends and cultures. But, of course, there is also the dark side-the risk of spending too much time online, the pressure to always show the best side of yourself, and the constant comparison with others.

And what about our addiction to the Internet? Before, we could live without it, but now it seems we can't help but check our e-mail, social media or the latest news every few minutes. It is as if we are become slaves of the digital world, always connected and always informed.

In short, smartphones and social media have changed our habits in ways we could never have imagined. We have become addicted to technology, always with our noses glued to the screen and always connected to the digital world. But at the same time, we also need to be aware of the risks and challenges this brings, and find a balance between the online and real worlds.

Concentration and Attention

let's talk about the effect that the inordinate use of technology has on our ability to concentrate. You know, it's like we've all become hyperactive bunnies, hopping from app to app without ever really stopping to focus on anything important.

Before, we could read a book for hours without distraction, or concentrate on a task without feeling tempted to check our phone every five minutes. But now? Well, we can't seem to concentrate on anything for more than a few minutes without feeling drawn in by a notification or a funny YouTube video.

And it is not only during our leisure time that the inordinate use of technology destroys our concentration. Even at work or school, it has become increasingly difficult to stay focused on complex or important tasks. It is as if our minds have become accustomed to jumping from one thing to another, without ever really stopping to think deeply.

And the problem is that this lack of concentration can have serious consequences on our daily lives. It can affect our work performance, our personal relationships and even our mental health. When we are unable to concentrate on one thing for a period of time prolonged period of time, we become more stressed, anxious and less productive.

In short, the inordinate use of technology certainly has an impact on our ability to concentrate. It is as if we have become addicted to the instant gratification that technology provides, and this has made it increasingly difficult for us to stay focused on one thing for an extended period of time. But at the same time, it is important to be aware of this problem and make a conscious effort to limit the use of technology when we need to focus on important tasks.

Let's talk about how we manage our attention in the digital world! It is like a constant battle between our desire to focus on something important and the endless distractions that surround us.

Before, we could sit and read a book without being interrupted by message notifications or alerts on social media. But now? Well, it seems we can't do a thing for more than two minutes without feeling tempted to check our phone to see if there is anything new happening in the digital world.

And what about multitasking? Before, we could focus on one task at a time and do it well. But now? Well, we seem to have become masters at doing a thousand things at once, jumping from one app to another without ever really completing anything.

But the problem is that this constant interruption of our attention has serious consequences on our ability to focus on important tasks. We become more stressed, less productive and more prone to make mistakes. It is as if the our mind had become a kind of battlefield, with distractions attacking us from all directions.

But, of course, all is not lost! We can learn to better manage our attention in the digital world.
We can set time limits for technology use, eliminate distracting notifications, and practice mindfulness to be more aware of the present moment. It is a challenge, but it is one we can take on, one notification at a time!

Learning and Memory

Shall we talk about how our beloved digital devices are affecting our learning? Get ready, because this is a real adventure into the world of bits and bytes!

First, let's take a look at how digital devices have changed the way we learn. Remember when you had to go to the library and flip through dozens of books to find the information you needed? Well, now all it takes is a quick Google search and voila, you have everything you need right there on your phone or computer screen!

But, of course, there is a downside. With the abundance of information available online, it becomes increasingly difficult to distinguish between what is true and what is false. It is as if we are swamped by a sea of news, and we have to do our best to navigate the waves of misinformation and find the dry land of truth.

But, in the end, all is not lost! We can learn to use our digital devices more consciously and responsibly. We can set time limits for technology use, eliminate digital distractions while studying, and use online tools to improve our learning. In short, with a little effort and determination, we can transform our digital devices from enemies of concentration into allies of learning!

Let's talk about how our faithful digital devices are affecting our ability to store information! It is as if we have all become goldfish, with a short-term memory that lasts only as long as a glance at our latest notification.

Before, we had to remember phone numbers, pin appointments on a paper calendar and study information for hours to memorize it. But now? Well, just a click and we can find any information we need on Google or Wikipedia. It's as if our brains have been tergiversating and refusing to remember things, knowing that technology can do it for us!

But there is more. With note-taking apps and the ability to save them to the cloud, we don't even have to worry about forgetting our brightest ideas. It's like having a personal digital assistant that keeps track of everything for us.
But, of course, there is a downside. Our dependence on these devices comes at a price, and we often find ourselves struggling to remember even the simplest things without our trusty phone at hand.

And what about our ability to concentrate? With digital distractions all around us, it becomes increasingly difficult to concentrate long enough to memorize new information. It is as if our attention has become an increasingly rare resource, and we must make a conscious effort to protect it from the assaults of notifications and social media.

In short, our digital devices have certainly made our lives easier in many ways, but they also have an impact on our ability to memorize information. It is as if we have become dependent on technology to remember things for us, and we have to make a conscious effort to exercise and keep our memory in shape.

Chapter 3: Mental Health

Let's talk about the effect that the inordinate use of technology has on our mental health. Get ready, because this is a descent into the darkness of our darkest thoughts!

Before, perhaps we were happier in ignorance. There wasn't the constant pressure to compare our lives with the perfect ones we see on social media, nor the constant anxiety of not being good enough or beautiful enough or interesting enough like others. But now? Well, it seems we can't escape from this race toward self-improvement and self-comparison, even though we know it's a losing battle from the start.

And what about addiction? It is as if we have become slaves to our devices, obsessively checking notifications and likes on social media as if they were our only glimmer of hope in an increasingly dark world. And when not enough likes or comments come in, we feel empty and unloved, as if our worth depends on the number of little hearts we receive.

But the worst is when we go down the rabbit hole of misinformation and online bias. With fake news spreading like wild fire on social media, it becomes increasingly difficult to distinguish between what is true and what is false. It is as if we are trapped in a maze of lies and conspiracies, with no way out and no hope of finding the truth.

And what about isolation? With technology keeping us constantly connected, it seems paradoxical that we feel increasingly lonely. Perhaps it is because our interactions have become so shallow and superficial that we feel empty and misunderstood, even when surrounded by thousands of online "friends."

In short, the inordinate use of technology has a devastating impact on our mental health. It makes us feel inadequate, lonely and even insane, as if we are trapped in a downward spiral of anxiety and depression. And even if we try to escape this digital prison, there seems to be no way out. What a beautiful perspective, isn't it? So let's face it: social media can be like a minefield for our mental health. It's as if there are traps hidden behind every like, comment or share.
When we don't get enough interactions or when we constantly compare ourselves to the perfect lives of others, that's when the cyclone of anxiety and depression begins.

Before, maybe we were a little more naive. There was not this constant pressure to show only the best of ourselves, to always appear happy and perfect in the eyes of others. But now? Well, it seems that we have all become masters at putting our lives on social media, even though behind those perfect photos is often a world of insecurities and discomforts.

And then there is the fake news and misinformation that spreads like a virus online. It is as if we are bombarded by an unceasing stream of bad news and conspiracy theories, fueling our anxiety and feeding our deepest fears. And even though we know that we cannot trust everything we read online, it is hard not to be swayed by all this negativism.

But the worst is when we get into the spiral of envy and jealousy. We look at the seemingly perfect lives of others and constantly compare ourselves with them, wondering why we cannot be as happy as they are. It is as if we are trapped in a golden cage of constant comparison, with no way out and no hope of finding true happiness.

In short, social media can be like a battleground for our mental health. It is as if we are constantly under siege by a series of invisible threats, threatening to plunge us further and further down the spiral of anxiety and depression. And even though we try to protect ourselves from it all, there always seems to be something new ready to pull us down into the abyss. What a situation, isn't it?

Okay, let's take a dive down the digital rabbit hole! Let's talk about our addiction to technology and how it is dragging us further and further down into the vortex of isolation and insecurity.

So let's take an honest look at our relationship with our devices. It's as if we are in a toxic relationship, where technology gives us that sense of comfort and connection, but at the same time keeps us captive in its digital grip. We find ourselves obsessively checking our phones, to look for that next shot of instant gratification that makes us feel temporarily better, even if it ultimately makes us feel empty and unsatisfied.

Before, perhaps we were more adept at balancing the digital and real worlds. But now? Well, we seem to be increasingly isolated, surrounded by bright screens that keep us company but at the same time keep us away from others.
It is as if we have become prisoners in our own home, trapped in the virtual world while the real world passes before our eyes.

And what about our self-esteem? With social media constantly showing us the perfect lives of others, it is easy to fall into the trap of constant comparison and feeling inadequate. It is as if we are all in a race to show who has the best life, even though a world of insecurities and hardships is often hidden behind those filtered photos.

But the worst is when we enter the vicious cycle of addiction and isolation. We find ourselves spending hours and hours online, isolated from the real world and surrounded by a false sense of connection. It is as if we are in an endless maze, where every time we think we find our way out, we only find ourselves returning to the starting point.

In short, our addiction to technology has become a digital prison that keeps us away from others and makes us feel increasingly lonely and insecure. And even as we try to escape from this prison, it seems that the chains of addiction are tightening around us. What a situation, isn't it?

Psychological mechanisms of addiction

When it comes to technology addiction, it is crucial to understand the underlying psychological mechanisms. Studies have shown that the immoderate use of technology can activate reward circuits in the brain, similar to those associated with substance abuse.
When we receive a notification or social confirmation on social media, our brains release neurotransmitters such as dopamine, which are involved in pleasure and gratification. This reinforces usage behavior and can lead to addiction.

In addition, excessive use of technology can negatively affect our ability to self-regulate and impulse control. When we are constantly immersed in digital devices, we may find it difficult to concentrate on tasks or activities that require patience and sustained attention. This can lead to a kind of "behavioral addiction," where we become dependent on the constant use of technology to meet our emotional and social needs.

At the same time, inordinate use of technology can negatively affect our mood and self-esteem. Social media, for example, constantly expose us to social comparisons and negative self-evaluations, which can contribute to the development of anxiety, depression and other mood disorders.

From a neurological perspective, constant exposure to the blue light emitted by digital device screens can affect our sleep-wake rhythm, interfering with melatonin production and disrupting our sleep. This can lead to sleep problems and fatigue, which in turn can negatively affect our mood, cognition and mental health.

In addition, addiction to technology can have negative effects on our ability to socialize and establish meaningful relationships in real life. When we spend too much time online, we may neglect face-to-face relationships and lose the ability to communicate effectively and empathetically with others.

In summary, technology addiction is a complex phenomenon involving a range of psychological, neurological, and social factors. Understanding these mechanisms can be critical to developing effective strategies to manage and reduce the inordinate use of technology and promote mental well-being.

Let's talk about how our daily lives have been transformed by the digital age! It is as if we have ended up on a continuous adventure, where we find ourselves navigating the challenges and conveniences of technology every day.

So, let's start with communication. Before, we had to wait days or even weeks to receive a response to a letter or call. But now? Well, all it takes is a text or video call and we can talk to anyone, anywhere they are in the world! It is as if the world has become a global village, connected by a maze of cables and electromagnetic waves.

And what about information? Before, we had to do endless research in books or encyclopedias to find answers to our questions. But now? Well, just a quick Google search and we can have an answer in seconds! It's like having access to an ocean of knowledge, all within reach of our fingers.

But there is also the dark side. With technology permeating every aspect of our lives, it has become increasingly difficult to disconnect and find a moment of peace and quiet. We are constantly bombarded with notifications, messages and digital stimuli that keep us connected 24/7. It is as if we are trapped in a digital cage, with no way out and no hope of finding true freedom.

And what about our mental health? With technology keeping us constantly connected and plugged in, it is easy to feel overwhelmed and overwhelmed. We are always connected, but we often feel more alone than ever before. It is as if we are all adrift in a sea of information, with no compass to guide us through the digital storms.

In short, our daily lives have been transformed by technology in ways we could never have imagined. It is as if we have gone on a wild adventure and unpredictable, where every day we find ourselves navigating the digital waves of modernity. What an exciting journey, isn't it?

Chapter 4: Interpersonal Relationships

let's talk about this epic battle between virtual and real communication! It is as if we have ended up in an arena where our old ways of communicating collide with new digital technologies.

So let's start with virtual communication. With the advent of smartphones and social media, it has become so easy to stay in touch with anyone, wherever they are.
We can send instant messages, make video calls, and share moments of our lives with the click of a button. It is as if the world has become a continuous party, with everyone connected and ready to communicate at all times.

But then there is real communication. The one face-to-face, with no filters or screens in between. That's the one that really makes you feel alive, when you can see the facial expressions and feel the emotions of the people around you. It's like we've gone back to our roots, when communication meant looking into each other's eyes and really listening to each other.

But herein lies the dilemma: which is better? Virtual communication offers us convenience and accessibility, but it lacks the human and authentic touch that only face-to-face communication can offer. It is as if we are torn between two worlds, trying to balance the convenience of technology with the desire for genuine connection.

And then there is the quality aspect of communication. With virtual communication, we are often bombarded with a series of messages and notifications, which can make it difficult to deepen conversations and truly understand others. It is as if we are trapped in a digital bedlam, where superficiality reigns supreme and authentic connection is a distant mirage.

But in the end, there is no right or wrong answer. Both types of communication have their advantages and disadvantages, and it is up to us as individuals to find a balance that works for us. Perhaps it is making time for coffee with a friend or a phone chat with a distant relative. Or maybe it's simply being aware of the way we use technology and making an effort to keep our face-to-face relationships alive. In the end, it's about finding that perfect mix of old and new, virtual and real, that makes us feel truly connected in today's world.

Let's dive into the difference between online and face-to-face interactions! It is like comparing two completely different worlds, each with its own charms and flaws.

So let's start with online interactions. When we talk on chat or social media, it is as if we have access to a universe of endless connections. We can chat with friends on the other side of the world, share moments from our life and discover new people with similar interests. It is like having a big virtual living room, where everyone is welcome and anything is possible.

But then there is the magic of face-to-face interactions. It's that tangible feeling of being truly present, seeing facial expressions and sensing the emotions of others. It is as if we are connected in a deeper way, truly understanding each other without the need for emoji or abbreviations.

But here's the difference: with online interactions, we have the advantage of convenience and speed. We can communicate instantly with anyone, wherever they are, without having to leave the comfort of our armchair. It is as if we have the whole world in our pocket, ready to be explored at the click of a button.

On the other hand, face-to-face interactions offer us a more authentic and deeper experience. We can truly connect with others, build meaningful relationships and create lasting memories. It is as if we have returned to our human roots, when communication meant looking into each other's eyes and truly listening to each other.

But in the end, both have their value. Online interactions offer us a world of opportunities and connections, while face-to-face interactions allow us to deepen relationships and experience the true essence of humanity. So why choose? Perhaps it is better to embrace both, finding a balance that allows us to enjoy the best of both worlds. Don't you think?

Effects on Social Skills

influence of technology on our social skills! It is as if we have ended up in a digital world where virtual communication is taking over from face-to-face interactions.

So let's start at the beginning. With the advent of smartphones and social media, our lives have become increasingly digital. We can communicate instantly with anyone, anywhere they are, without having to lift a single finger. It is as if we are all connected in one big virtual network, where relationships are formed and developed through bright screens.

But there is a cost to be paid. With most of our interactions taking place online, we risk losing sight of the importance of social skills in the real world. It is as if we have become dependent on technology to communicate with others, forgetting the art of listening, making eye contact and interpreting facial expressions.

This is why it is so important to balance our online interactions with face-to-face interactions. Social skills are essential for building meaningful relationships, managing conflict, and navigate the real world. It is as if they are the foundation on which our emotional and social well-being is based.

But how can we cultivate these skills in an era dominated by technology? Well, we can start by practicing mindfulness. Let's take the time to take our eyes off the screen and look at the world around us. Let's really listen to others and try to understand their perspectives. It's like going back to the basics of human interaction, where connection is created through mutual understanding and empathy.

In addition, we can take advantage of the opportunities offered by technology to improve our social skills. We can participate in online forums, attend interest groups and participate in virtual events to practice the art of conversation and collaboration. It is like being in a virtual boot camp, where we can practice and hone our social skills in a controlled environment.

In short, the influence of technology on our social skills is a complex and ever-changing topic. But with awareness, practice and a little balance, we can find a way to navigate between the virtual and real worlds and cultivate meaningful relationships that enrich our lives.

Influences on sociality

Here we are talking about how technology is affecting our social skills! It's a topic I'm really passionate about, so hang in there as we explore this digital world together.

So let's start with the basics. With all these digital devices and social media, it seems that we are always connected, but at the same time more distant than ever. It's as if we are surrounded by a sea of notifications and messages, but missing those real moments of human connection.

Here's the dilemma: while technology offers us a myriad of ways to communicate, we risk losing sight of basic social skills. It's as if we've all become masters of rapid keystroke typing, but no longer know how to have an interesting conversation over a cup of coffee.

But all is not lost! We can do something to keep our social skills alive even in an increasingly digital world. For example, we can set aside our phones and make an effort to meet friends in person. It's like going back to the roots of humanity, where relationships were built around a fire, not a WhatsApp group.

In addition, we can be more aware of how we use technology in our social interactions. Instead of just exchanging quick messages, we can make an effort to really listen to others and respond in a meaningful way. It is as if we go back to the old school of communication, where words had a deeper weight and meaning.

Finally, we can harness the power of technology to cultivate meaningful relationships. We can participate in online groups that share our interests, attend virtual events, or even make new friends through social platforms. It is as if we are in a vast digital universe, full of possibilities for connection and discovery.

In short, technology can be a double-edged sword when it comes to our social skills, but with a little awareness and effort we can find a balance that allows us to keep human relationships alive in an increasingly digital world.

Influence on social dynamics

here is an interesting topic: the changes in social dynamics caused by technology! It is as if we are on a mad dash through a digital amusement park, where each turn and corner takes us into new and uncharted territory of our human interactions.

So let's start with the obvious: technology has revolutionized the way we connect with others. With smartphones, social media and instant messaging apps, we are always connected, even if we are physically far away. It is as if the whole world has become our backyard, with the possibility of meeting people and making friends in every corner of the globe.

But there is a downside. While technology offers us an unprecedented network of connections, we risk losing sight of the quality of our interactions. It is as if we have become adept at maintaining superficial contact with hundreds of people online, but lack the deep and meaningful connections that only face-to-face relationships can provide.

In addition, technology has introduced new forms of communication and expression. We have emoji, stickers, GIFs and memes to communicate our emotions and thoughts quickly and entertainingly. It is as if we are in a world of symbolic languages, where a smiley face can say more than a thousand words.

But what happens to our "traditional" social skills? With so much time spent behind screens, we risk becoming awkward or insecure about face-to-face interactions. It is as if we have become masters in the art of digital communication, but we lack the ability to read the nuances of a smile or a handshake.

In short, technology has brought momentous changes to our social dynamics. It has given us a world of possibilities, but it has also confronted us with new challenges and dilemmas. But in the end, it is up to us as individuals to find a balance that allows us to successfully navigate the ever-widening sea of our human relationships.

Chapter 5: Online Safety and Cyberbullying

Let's dig into the darkness of the web and see what emerges! Let's talk about the dangers behind every click and every like.

So, the online world may seem like an endless playground, but there is a dark area we have to face: the dangers of the Web. It is as if there are traps hidden behind every site and every profile we visit.

First of all, there is the privacy risk. We share so much personal information online, from our photos to our addresses, without even realizing the consequences. It is as if we are opening the door of our house to anyone who wants to enter, without knowing who might be on the other side.

Then there is cyberbullying, a real scourge of the digital world. It is as if there is an army of bullies hiding behind every screen, ready to target anyone who stands in their way. Victims can be deeply hurt from cruel words and online attacks, leaving emotional scars that can last for years.

And let's not forget the sexual predators who hide behind fake online profiles, trying to lure young people into their web. It's like a dangerous game of cat and mouse, with potentially disastrous consequences for innocent victims.

But how can we protect ourselves from these dangers? It is as if we need to arm ourselves with awareness and caution. Learning how to protect our privacy online, avoid sharing sensitive information, and being aware of potential risks is a good place to start.

In addition, we need to be ready to intervene when we see someone being cyberbullied or to lend a hand to anyone who is struggling online. It is as if we need to create a virtual support network, ready to extend a helping hand to anyone in need.

In short, the Web can be a wonderful place, but there are hidden potholes along the way. It is as if we must learn to navigate these dangerous waters wisely and cautiously, to protect ourselves and those around us.

let's face the monster of cyberbullying! It is as if there is a real digital dragon ready to devour the self-esteem and happiness of anyone in its path.

So, cyberbullying is like traditional bullying, but with a digital twist. It involves attacks, insults or threats that occur online, through social media, instant messages or other digital platforms. It is as if bullies have found a new battleground where they can hide behind the screen and attack their victims mercilessly.

And the damage can be devastating. Victims of cyberbullying can feel isolated, humiliated and helpless in the face of constant attacks. It is as if they are trapped in a digital nightmare, with no way out and no one to turn to for help.

But the scary thing is that cyberbullying can follow victims wherever they go, thanks to the pervasive nature of technology. It is as if there is no safe haven, no corner of the digital world where they can feel safe.

But what can we do to combat this digital monster? Well, it's like we need to join forces to create a safer and more respectful online environment for everyone. We can intervene when we see someone being cyberbullied, offering support and solidarity. We can also report abusive behavior to online platforms and relevant authorities.

In addition, it is important to educate young people about the consequences of cyberbullying and how to protect themselves online. It is as if we need to arm people with the awareness and skills to defend themselves against digital attacks.

In short, cyberbullying is like a monster lurking in the web's meanders, but we can defeat it together with courage, solidarity and awareness. It is as if we have to be the digital heroes fighting for a safer and more respectful online world for all.

Online predators

online predators, the terror of the darkest corners of the web! It is as if there is a pack of dire wolves lurking, ready to target anyone in their digital territory.

So, these predators are like masters of deception, disguised behind false profiles and identities. They can pretend to be anyone, from harmless girls next door to handsome guys, to lure their victims into a trap. It is as if they are true deception artists, ready to play with people's emotions and vulnerabilities.

And their victims? They are often young, naive and vulnerable, easily swayed by the flattery and promises of predators. It is as if they were hungry fish bitten by the hook, not realizing the danger that awaits them beneath the surface.

But what do these online predators seek? Well, it is usually a combination of power, control, and sexual gratification. It is as if they are hunters looking for their prey, ready to exploit any weakness to get what they want.

And the damage can be devastating. Victims can be subjected to harassment, blackmail, sexual abuse, and even online exploitation. It is as if they are trapped in a maze of digital terror, with no way out and no one to turn to for help.

But can we fight these online predators? Absolutely we can! It is as if we have to be true digital warriors, ready to protect ourselves and others from the danger behind the screen. We can educate young people about online safety, teaching them to recognize the warning signs and protect themselves from online threats. And we can also report suspicious behavior to the appropriate authorities to ensure that predators are brought to justice.

In short, online predators are like dark shadows in the digital world, but we can illuminate these dark corners with awareness, vigilance and action. It is as if we are supposed to be the light that drives out the darkness, protecting anyone in our digital territory.

Cybersecurity

Now let's start with viruses and malware. It is as if there are little digital monsters lurking around waiting to infect our devices. They can steal our personal information, damage our files or even take complete control of our computer. It is as if we are in a constant battle against an army of malevolent creatures trying to invade our digital world.

And then there are the online scams. It is as if there are masters of deception who try to trick people into stealing money or sensitive information from them. They may pretend to be financial institutions, legitimate businesses or even friends in trouble, trying to gain access to our bank accounts or passwords. It is as if we should always be on guard, ready to challenge any offer that is too good to be true.

And let's not forget the dark side of social media. It is as if there is a valley of trolls and haters, ready to sow discord and hatred in every post and comment. They can intimidate, threaten or defame others, creating a toxic and damaging climate for the online community. It is as if we must always keep our digital sword drawn, ready to defend ourselves and others from these evil forces.

In short, the Internet can be a wonderful place, but there are also dangers waiting for us behind every click. It is as if we have to be true digital explorers, ready to navigate through this digital jungle with caution, wisdom and awareness.

Prevention and Protection Strategies

How to defend ourselves against these dangers! It is as if we have to be real digital ninjas, ready to take on any threat that lurks behind a screen.

So, let's start with viruses and malware. To protect ourselves from these little digital fiends, we can arm our devices with antivirus and antispyware software. It is as if we put an armor around our data, ready to fend off any digital attack that is thrown at us.

When it comes to online scams, we need to be as cunning as foxes. We have to learn to recognize the most common scams, such as phishing schemes or too-good-to-be-true offers. It is as if we have to train our senses to spot every hidden trap in the digital world.

And as for social media, we can defend ourselves by creating a circle of trust around us. It is like building a castle with thick walls, ready to protect us from the poisonous arrows of haters and trolls. We can also

Learn how to manage privacy settings to control who can see our information and posts.

But the most powerful defense is education. It is as if we are armed with knowledge to fight every threat that comes our way. We need to educate ourselves and others about the dangers of the web, teaching them how to recognize and avoid digital traps. It is as if we spread the light of awareness to every dark corner of the web.

In short, we can fight these digital dangers, but we have to be ready to bring all our resources and ingenuity to bear. It is as if we are in a great digital battle, ready to defend ourselves and others from every threat that awaits us in the online world.

it is as if we are grappling with a real superhero mission: to protect young people from the dark dangers that lurk in the digital world. So let's set out to find all the weapons and strategies we can use to fight this battle!

To begin with, we need to educate young people about the dangers of the Web. It is as if we have to sit them in the front row and tell them about all the pitfalls they can encounter online, from scams to sexual predators. We need to make them understand that the Web can be a wonderful place, but there are also dark areas they need to avoid.

But it is not enough just to warn them, we must also provide them with the tools to defend themselves. It is as if we are arming young people with a belt of digital tools, ready to deal with every threat that arises. We need to teach them how to recognize scams, protect their online privacy, and manage their security settings on social media.

And let's not forget about open communication and support. It's like we need to be like a bulwark, ready to listen and support young people at all times. We need to encourage them to talk to us if something is wrong or if they feel uncomfortable online. It is important that they feel free to share their concerns without fear of being judged.

In addition, we need to team up with schools, authorities and local organizations to create a safe online environment for young people. It is as if we have to join forces and resources to create educational programs, promote online safety, and ensure that there are resources available for those who need them.

Finally, we need to be positive role models for young people. It is as if we should be beacons of light in the dark, showing them how to navigate the web responsibly and respectfully. We need to be aware of our own online actions and show them that it is possible to enjoy the benefits of the web without falling into the traps of its dangers.

In short, protecting young people from the dangers of the Web is a challenging mission, but with commitment, awareness and support we can make a difference. It is as if we are a team of superheroes ready to fight for a safer and more secure digital world for all.

Safety behaviors

Let's dig deeper into this! Promoting safe online behaviors is like planting the foundation for a healthy and protected digital environment for all. And to do this best, we must be prepared to explore every aspect of this mission.

First, we need to educate young people about the risks and threats that lurk on the Web. It is as if we have to create a complete digital instruction manual, with all the information they need to navigate safely online. We need to teach them how to recognize scams, protect their privacy, avoid cyberbullying, and deal with sexual predators. Every detail is important, because even the smallest knowledge can make a difference when it comes to online safety.

But it is not enough just to tell them what to do, we must also show them by example. It is as if we have to be true digital pioneers, ready to show others the way to safe web surfing. We need to be aware of our actions online, avoiding risky or irresponsible behavior that could put ourselves or others in danger. After all, we are the role models for young people, and our online conduct can have a significant impact on their actions and choices.

In addition, we need to provide them with the tools and resources they need to safely navigate the digital world. It's like we need to be like a digital defense arsenal, with anti-virus software, protection filters, and tools to manage security on social media. We need to teach them how to use these resources effectively and responsibly so that they can protect themselves from online dangers.

But promoting online safety is not just about young people, it's about all of us. It's like we need to create a culture of digital safety, where everyone feels responsible for their own safety and the safety of others.
We need to encourage the sharing of information and resources on online safety, promoting greater awareness and understanding of risks and best practices to protect ourselves.

Finally, we must be ready to evolve and adapt to changes in the digital landscape. It is as if we have to be like real digital detectives, always one step ahead of new dangers and threats that emerge.
We must be ready to provide up-to-date information and innovative solutions to address emerging problems in the ever-changing digital world.

In short, promoting safe online behavior is a complex and multifaceted mission that requires commitment, knowledge and cooperation from everyone. But with a comprehensive and proactive approach, we can make a difference in creating a safer and more secure digital environment for all.

Chapter 6: Technology and Education

the educational advantages of the web! It is as if we are facing a vast ocean of knowledge, with endless resources and learning opportunities just a click away. And this ocean is not only a source of information, but also a true interactive learning laboratory, where young people can explore, discover and create in ways never seen before.

First of all, the Web offers unprecedented access to knowledge. It is as if there were an endless library available to everyone, where information on any topic imaginable can be found. From literary classics to the latest scientific discoveries, everything is just a click away for anyone with access to the Internet.

But it is not only the quantity of information that matters, it is also the variety and quality. It is as if there is a wide range of online resources, from academic texts to video lectures, from interactive simulations to forum discussions. This diversity of formats and approaches makes online learning more engaging and accessible for a wide range of learners.

In addition, the Web offers the opportunity for personalized and adaptive learning. It is as if there is a virtual tutor who follows students step by step along their learning path, adapting the material and activities according to their needs and abilities. This personalized approach can help students overcome their challenges and develop their skills more effectively.

But the educational benefits of the Web do not stop there. It is as if there is an entire online learning community where students can connect and collaborate with others from all over the world. Through discussion forums, online study groups and collaborative projects, students can share ideas, solve problems and learn from each other in a stimulating and inclusive virtual environment.

In addition, the Web offers a range of tools and resources for hands-on, experience-based learning. It is as if there are virtual labs, interactive simulations, and content creation platforms that allow students to experience and apply what they have learned in tangible and meaningful ways.

In short, the educational benefits of the web are vast and diverse, offering students an unprecedented opportunity to access knowledge, interact with others, and develop their skills creatively and authentically. It is as if the web has become a true global campus, where learning has no boundaries or limits.

Integrating technology to education

The integration of technology in education offers a number of benefits that go far beyond simply digitizing learning materials. It is as if we are facing a real paradigm shift in learning, with the potential to radically transform the educational experience for students of all ages.

First, technology offers unprecedented access to knowledge and educational resources. It is as if there were a vast treasure trove of information just a click away, available 24/7 from anywhere in the world. This unlimited access allows students to explore topics in depth, deepen their understanding, and access high-quality educational materials, regardless of their geographic location or available resources.

But it is not only a matter of quantity, it is also a matter of quality. It is as if technology offers us a wide range of interactive tools and resources that make learning more engaging, dynamic and personalized. From instructional videos to interactive simulations, from the multimedia presentations to online learning platforms, students have access to a variety of learning modes that suit their individual style and specific needs.

In addition, technology offers new opportunities for collaboration and communication. It is as if there is a virtual bridge connecting students and teachers around the world, enabling them to share ideas, collaborate on projects, and learn from each other in a stimulating and inclusive digital environment. Through discussion forums, video conferencing and online collaboration platforms, students can develop communication and collaboration skills essential for success in the modern world.

But perhaps one of the greatest benefits of integrating technology into education is its ability to make learning more accessible and inclusive for all students. It is as if technology removes the physical and cognitive barriers that can hinder traditional learning, offering tools and resources that can be tailored to the individual needs of students with disabilities or special needs. Through screen-reading software, machine translation programs, and other assistive technologies, students can access the curriculum and fully participate in the educational experience, regardless of their abilities or challenges.

In short, integrating technology into education offers a number of benefits that go far beyond simply digitizing learning materials. It is as if we are moving toward a new way of learning, where technology is not just a tool, but a resource

Essential for the enrichment and innovation of the educational experience

Tools suitable for learning

Let's talk about digital tools for learning, which represent a real revolution in the world of education. It is as if we are faced with a vast arsenal of resources and technologies that can radically transform the way students learn and interact with learning materials.

First, let's talk about educational software. It is as if there is a wide range of programs designed specifically to support student learning. These software programs can cover a wide range of topics, from math to language to science to history, offering interactive lessons, hands-on exercises and assessment tools to help students develop their skills in an effective and engaging way.

But it is not just a matter of pre-packaged software, it is also a matter of flexible and customizable digital tools. It is as if there is a wide range of online tools and resources that enable teachers to create customized learning materials tailored to the specific needs of their students. From multimedia presentations to interactive teaching sheets, from online quizzes to gamification activities, teachers have a wide range of tools at their disposal to meet their students' individual needs and support them in their learning journey.

Also, let's talk about online learning platforms. It is as if there is a whole digital ecosystem dedicated to education, where students can access courses, lectures and educational resources from anywhere in the world.
These platforms offer a variety of courses on a wide range of topics, allowing students to deepen their interests and develop new skills independently and flexibly.

But perhaps one of the greatest benefits of digital tools for learning is their ability to foster collaboration and communication among students. It is as if there are virtual bridges connecting students around the world, enabling them to share ideas, solve problems and work together on common projects. Through discussion forums, online study groups and digital collaboration tools, students can learn from each other in an inclusive and stimulating environment.

In short, digital tools for learning offer an unprecedented opportunity to transform the educational experience for students. It is as if we are in a new era of education, where technology is a powerful ally to enrich and enhance the learning process for all.

Disadvantages and Distractions

we explore more deeply the challenges associated with the use of technology in educational settings. Although technology offers many benefits in education, it is also important to recognize and address the challenges and complexities it brings.

A major challenge is the need to ensure equity in access to technology. Not all students have access to reliable digital devices or stable internet connections at home, which can create inequalities in access to online educational resources. It is as if there is a digital divide that can widen existing disparities among students from different socioeconomic backgrounds.
Addressing this challenge requires a commitment from educational institutions and policymakers to ensure that all students have access to the tools and resources they need to learn effectively.

Another challenge is distraction and technology addiction. It is as if we are grappling with a constant struggle to keep students' attention focused on learning, while being bombarded by notifications, messages and other digital distractions. In addition, overuse of technology can lead to screen addiction, with potential negative effects on students' mental health and well-being. Addressing this challenge requires a combination of educational strategies, such as teaching time management and concentration skills, along with school and family policies that promote balanced use of technology.

Another element to consider is the privacy and security of student data. With the increased use of technology in classrooms, there is a growing concern about the collection, storage and use of students' personal data by digital platforms and educational applications. It is as if there is a risk of privacy breaches and misuse of data, which could put students' safety and well-being at risk. Addressing this challenge requires strict policies on data protection and student privacy, along with increased awareness and training for teachers and students themselves on the importance of online safety.

Finally, there is the challenge of effectively integrating technology into teaching and learning. It is as if there is a need to develop digital skills among teachers so that they can effectively use digital tools and resources to support student learning. In addition, it is important to ensure that the use of technology is pedagogically sound and aimed at enhancing student learning, rather than simply being an ancillary addition to traditional teaching activities.

In short, the challenges related to the use of technology in educational settings are complex and multifaceted. It is as if we must address these challenges with a holistic approach, combining policies, practices, and resources that promote responsible, equitable, and effective use of technology to support student learning

Technological distractions

the issue of technological distractions in the classroom. With the increased use of digital devices among students, it has become increasingly difficult to maintain focused attention on learning without being disturbed by notifications, messages or other digital distractions.

One of the main challenges related to technological distractions is their impact on students' concentration and learning. It is as if we are immersed in a world where students are constantly tempted to check their devices for messages, social media updates, or other notifications, instead of focusing on classroom learning activities. This constant interruption can impair students' ability to maintain attention and fully engage in learning activities, negatively affecting their academic performance and long-term success.

In addition, technological distractions can also have an impact on classroom dynamics and the overall learning climate. It is as if there is a kind of fracture in group cohesion, with some students being completely immersed in their devices while others are trying to to stay focused on classroom activities. This discrepancy can create tension and discomfort among students and with the teacher, compromising the effectiveness of the learning environment and hindering collaboration and interaction among students.

In addition, technological distractions can also impact students' mental health and well-being. It is as if we are facing a kind of cognitive overload, with students constantly bombarded with digital stimuli that can cause stress, anxiety and mental fatigue. This can lead to a decrease in students' satisfaction and well-being, compromising their motivation and engagement in learning.

Addressing technology distractions in the classroom requires a holistic, multilevel approach. It is as if we must adopt a combination of instructional strategies, school policies, and individual support to help students effectively manage their technology use habits and keep their attention focused on learning.

This may include implementing school policies that regulate the use of digital devices in the classroom, establishing specific times for use and banning during class, as well as educating students on healthy and responsible technology use habits. It is like educating students about the potential negative effects of technological distractions and providing them with strategies and tools to effectively manage digital temptations and keep their attention focused on learning.

In addition, it is important to create a stimulating and engaging learning environment that takes into account the needs and of students' interests, minimizing opportunities for boredom and disengagement that can lead to technological distractions. It is as if we should adopt active and participatory teaching approaches that actively engage students in learning and motivate them to participate fully in classroom activities.

Finally, it is important to involve students in the educational process, allowing them to actively participate in setting rules and expectations for technology use in the classroom and to collaborate with teachers and other students to find effective solutions to technological distractions. It is as if we need to create a sense of shared responsibility and collective commitment to maintain a focused and productive learning environment for all students.

Chapter 7: Solutions and Recommendations

Addressing the challenge of digital education comprehensively requires a detailed overview of its many dimensions and implications. First and foremost, it is important to understand that digital education is not limited to the use of technology in teaching and learning, but embraces a broader approach involving the development of digital skills that are fundamental to meeting the challenges and taking advantage of the opportunities of the digital society.

One of the main dimensions of digital education is the development of digital skills among students. It is akin to ensuring that students acquire the knowledge and skills needed to use technology effectively and responsibly in a variety of contexts, from online research activities to digital communication, from creating digital content to protecting online privacy. This also includes critical awareness and the ability to critically evaluate online information, distinguishing between reliable and unreliable sources, and understanding the ethical and legal implications of using technology.

In addition, digital education also includes promoting digital inclusion, ensuring that all students have access to resources and opportunities provided by technology. It is like we need to address inequalities in access to technology and ensure that students from disadvantaged socio-economic backgrounds or with disabilities have the same learning opportunities as those from more privileged backgrounds. This can include access to digital devices and reliable internet connections, as well as training and support to effectively use digital tools for learning.

In addition, digital education also includes promoting digital citizenship and online safety. It is as if we are faced with the need to educate students about the risks and threats associated with the use of technology, such as cyberbullying, phishing, and identity theft, and provide them with the skills and strategies to protect themselves from these threats and navigate the digital world safely and responsibly.
This also includes promoting ethical and responsible behavior online, such as respecting the privacy of others, being kind online, and complying with data protection laws and regulations.

Finally, digital education also includes promoting innovation and creativity through the use of technology. It is like we should encourage students to experiment, explore and create using digital tools, encouraging their curiosity and innovative spirit. This can include technology-based learning projects, such as creating blogs, podcasts, videos or other digital content, which allow students to express their ideas and knowledge in creative and authentic ways.

In summary, digital education is a broad and complex concept that goes beyond the simple use of technology in teaching and learning. It is as if we are faced with the need to develop a holistic approach that embraces the promotion of digital skills, digital inclusion, digital citizenship, and digital creativity among students, ensuring that they are ready to meet the challenges and take advantage of the opportunities of the digital society in which we live.

The importance of education for conscious use.

We explore in detail the importance of teaching informed and critical use of technology. This topic is of paramount importance in the digital age in which we live, as technology has become an integral part of daily life and profoundly influences the way we live, work and learn.

First, teaching informed use of technology is crucial to helping individuals understand the role and impact of technology in their lives. It is as if we are faced with the need to educate individuals about the benefits and challenges associated with the use of technology, as well as the social, cultural and ethical implications of it.
This includes awareness of the risks associated with online privacy and security, as well as understanding the implications of technology on mental health, interpersonal relationships and general well-being.

Second, teaching critical use of technology is essential for developing individuals' cognitive and analytical skills. It is as if we should encourage individuals to critically evaluate the information they find online, distinguishing between reliable and unreliable sources and understanding how information is manipulated and presented through digital media. This includes.

also the ability to recognize and counter misinformation and fake news, promoting a culture of critical and analytical thinking that is fundamental to active and informed participation in contemporary society.

In addition, teaching informed and critical use of technology can help mitigate the risks associated with overuse or misuse of technology. It is like educating individuals about the potential negative effects of overuse of technology on mental health, interpersonal relationships, and overall well-being, as well as the strategies and resources available to effectively manage technology use and maintain a healthy balance between online and offline life.

Finally, teaching informed and critical use of technology can promote active and responsible participation in digital society. It is as if we should encourage individuals to use technology creatively and constructively to contribute to problem solving and community improvement. This also includes promoting ethical and responsible online behaviors, such as respecting the privacy of others, complying with data protection laws and regulations, and adhering to online norms of behavior.

In summary, teaching informed and critical use of technology is essential to prepare individuals to effectively and responsibly navigate the digital society in which we live. It is as if we must provide them with the knowledge, skills, and resources they need to use technology safely, intelligently, and ethically, promoting active and informed participation in contemporary society.

Literacy programs

Let us examine in detail the importance of digital literacy programs and their impact in contemporary society. Digital literacy is not simply limited to knowing how to use a computer or navigate the Internet, but encompasses a set of fundamental skills needed to participate fully and responsibly in digital society.

First and foremost, digital literacy programs are essential to bridging the digital divide. In an age when technology has become ubiquitous and many aspects of daily life are digitized, it is critical to ensure that everyone has access and skills to use technology effectively. This is especially important for individuals from disadvantaged socio-economic backgrounds or with disabilities, who may otherwise risk being excluded from the opportunities offered by the digital society.

In addition, digital literacy programs are crucial to promoting digital inclusion. They are not only about providing individuals with access to Internet devices and connections, but also ensuring that they have the skills needed to use technology effectively and meaningfully. This includes the ability to search for information online, communicate effectively through digital means, and use digital tools to solve problems and achieve personal and professional goals.

In addition, digital literacy programs are essential to prepare individuals for the world of work. As the economy becomes increasingly digitized, more and more jobs require fundamental digital skills, such as the ability to use productivity software, communicate through digital means and adapt quickly to technological changes. Digital literacy programs can provide individuals with the skills they need to succeed in the contemporary job market and access rewarding, well-paying employment opportunities.

In addition, digital literacy programs can help improve civic participation and political awareness. With the increased use of technology in decision-making and governance, it is important that individuals have the skills necessary to understand and participate effectively in political and civic life. This includes the ability to critically evaluate online information, participate in public debates through social media, and use digital tools to defend their rights and interests.

Finally, digital literacy programs can help promote online safety and security. With the rise of cybersecurity threats such as phishing, malware, and identity theft, it is critical that individuals are aware of the risks and strategies to protect their privacy and security online. Digital literacy programs can provide individuals with the knowledge and skills needed to recognize and address these threats effectively.

In conclusion, digital literacy programs are essential to empower individuals to participate fully and responsibly in the digital society. By equipping individuals with the skills needed to use technology effectively, these programs can help bridge the digital divide, promote digital inclusion, prepare individuals for the world of work, enhance civic participation, and promote online safety.

Methods of approach

Addressing parents' needs in using technology requires a detailed and sensitive approach to their challenges and needs. Here are some key aspects to consider:

Technology Education: Parents can benefit from educational programs designed to teach them how to use technology effectively and support their children in the digital environment in which we live. This could include workshops on online safety, managing time spent in front of screens, and best practices for family digital communication.

Supervision and Monitoring Strategies: It is important to provide parents with the tools and strategies they need to supervise their children's online activity responsibly. This could involve using parental control software, monitoring social media activity, and openly communicating with their children about their online experiences.

Promoting Open Conversation: Open communication between parents and children about the use of technology is crucial. Encouraging parents to establish open dialogues with their children can help them feel more comfortable sharing their experiences online and addressing any problems.

Behavior Models: Parents play a crucial role as role models for their children. By using technology in a balanced and responsible way, they can show their children how to use technology in a healthy and productive way.

Family Communication and Limits: Open family communication is essential to establish clear limits on technology use in the home. Parents should work with their children to set rules and limits on the use of digital devices, including time limits and rules on privacy and online safety.

Continuing Education: Parents should have access to continuing education opportunities on the evolution of technology and the new risks and opportunities it brings. This could include information sessions, webinars, and online resources to help them stay up-to-date on the latest trends and best practices in family technology use.

Support Resources: Making support resources available to parents, such as online guidelines, parent support groups, and counseling services, can be of great help in dealing with the challenges of using technology and getting advice and support from experts.

In summary, providing support to parents in their use of technology requires a comprehensive approach that includes education, communication, supervision, and access to supportive resources. Helping parents navigate the rapidly changing digital world can help ensure that families are able to meet the challenges and take advantage of the opportunities of the digital society responsibly.

Role of teachers

When it comes to the role of teachers and educational institutions in digital education, it is important to consider a number of detailed aspects that reflect the challenges and opportunities that arise in an increasingly digitized world.

Teachers play a crucial role in integrating technology into the learning environment. This means not only understanding the digital tools available, but also using them creatively to enrich students' learning experience. Ongoing training is essential to ensure that teachers keep their digital skills up-to-date and are able to effectively use digital tools in their teaching.

In addition to using technology to enhance teaching and learning, teachers must also promote critical thinking and media literacy among students. This means teaching them how to critically evaluate online information, recognize misinformation, and understand the social, cultural, and ethical implications of using technology.

Educational institutions play a key role in supporting teachers and ensuring that they are able to use technology effectively. This includes providing them with resources and technical support, as well as developing clear policies and guidelines on the use of technology in the classroom. These policies need to address important issues such as online safety, student privacy, and accessibility of digital resources.

In addition, educational institutions should actively collaborate with families and the community to promote responsible and aware use of technology. This may involve holding informational meetings for parents, online safety workshops for students, and partnerships with local organizations to promote digital literacy and online safety in the broader community.

Finally, it is important for educational institutions to regularly assess the impact of technology use on student learning and well-being. This could include collecting data on the effectiveness of digital resources used in the classroom, monitoring time spent in front of screens, and assessing students' online safety and privacy.

In summary, both teachers and educational institutions play a key role in students' digital education.
By providing training, resources and support, they can help students develop the skills they need to succeed in an increasingly digitized world.

Chapter 8: Conclusions

When considering the role of teachers and educational institutions in digital education, a number of essential considerations emerge that reflect the challenges and opportunities of an increasingly technology-driven world.

Teachers, in particular, must be prepared to transform themselves from mere transmitters of knowledge to facilitators of learning. This requires not only a mastery of the available technological means, but also a thorough understanding of how to use these tools to stimulate students' creativity, critical thinking and collaboration.

Educational institutions must play an active role in supporting teachers in this transformation process. This includes providing resources, training and technical support to help teachers effectively integrate technology into teaching and learning. In addition, educational institutions must develop clear policies and guidelines on the use of technology in the classroom, ensuring that crucial issues such as online safety, student privacy, and accessibility of digital resources are addressed.

It is also important to actively involve families and the community in the digital education process. Families can play a key role in supporting students in the responsible use of technology at home, while collaboration with the community can provide additional learning opportunities and resources for students.

In addition, it is important to ensure that digital education is equitable and inclusive for all students. This means addressing the digital divide and provide additional support to students from disadvantaged socio-economic backgrounds or with disabilities, ensuring that they have equitable access to digital resources and learning opportunities.

In conclusion, teachers and educational institutions play a crucial role in educating students for an increasingly digital world. By supporting teachers, engaging families and the community, and promoting equity and inclusion, we can ensure that all students have the skills they need to succeed in an increasingly technology-driven global economy.

In the context of digital education, there is room for an optimistic view of the future as numerous advances and opportunities emerge that offer hope for the improvement of students' educational experience.

One of the main findings emerging is the transformative potential of technology in learning. Digital tools offer the possibility of personalizing learning for students, tailoring lessons to their individual needs and learning styles. This means that teachers can create more engaging and meaningful learning experiences that motivate students to explore and deepen their interests.

In addition, technology opens the door to new forms of collaboration and knowledge sharing. Students can connect with their peers around the world, collaborate on shared projects and access a wide range of educational resources online. This greatly expands their prospects and prepares them for a globalized and interconnected world.

Another promising aspect is the role of artificial intelligence in education. With AI, it is possible to develop intelligent learning systems that provide personalized feedback to students and guide them through the learning process more effectively. This means that teachers can focus on value-added activities, such as guiding and providing personalized support to students, while AI takes care of the more repetitive and routine tasks.

In addition, digital education offers new opportunities to address the educational gap and promote equity in education. Digital resources can be easily accessible to all students, regardless of their geographic location or socioeconomic background. This means that even students from disadvantaged communities can access the same learning opportunities as those from more privileged backgrounds.

Finally, there is the positive impact that digital education can have on students' development of 21st century skills to consider. Working with technology not only improves their technical skills, but also soft skills such as problem solving, creativity, and collaboration. These skills are essential to prepare students for the world of work of the future, which requires flexibility, adaptability and critical thinking skills.

In conclusion, despite the challenges that digital education may present, there are numerous findings that offer hope and promise to positively transform the educational experience of students. With the efforts of the teachers, the support of educational institutions and the responsible adoption of technology, we can look to the future with optimism and confidence in the potential of technology to improve education for all.

Future Perspectives

Looking to the future of digital education opens up vast and fascinating horizons that promise to radically transform the way we learn and teach.

The advent of artificial intelligence opens the door to more personalized and targeted learning. Imagine a future where students can benefit from tailored teaching, where content is tailored to their specific needs and feedback is immediate and personalized. AI could help teachers identify each student's strengths and areas for improvement, allowing them to intervene in a timely and targeted manner.

At the same time, virtual and augmented reality open up extraordinary possibilities for immersion and sensory experience. Imagine being able to explore Egyptian pyramids or examine human body cells up close, all without leaving your classroom. Technology can transform learning from a passive to a participatory and immersive experience, fueling students' curiosity and enthusiasm.

Increasing global connectivity also offers unprecedented opportunities for collaboration and knowledge exchange. Students can connect with their peers around the world, share projects and ideas, and learn from each other. This global dimension of learning not only promotes diversity and inclusion, but also prepares students for an increasingly interconnected and intercultural world.

However, as we embrace these new technologies, it is important to remember to maintain an ethical and responsible approach. We must be mindful of the social and cultural impacts of our technology choices, and work to ensure that access to digital education is equitable and inclusive for all students, regardless of their background or circumstances.

In conclusion, the future of digital education is full of possibilities and promise. With the smart and informed use of technology, we can transform learning into an engaging, meaningful and inclusive experience, preparing students to meet the challenges and seize the opportunities of tomorrow's world.

Impact on the next generation

When we consider the impact of digital education on future generations, we enter territory rich in possibilities and challenges, where the prospects are broad and the changing landscape of the digital world opens unprecedented horizons.

Looking to the future, we see an educational environment where technology is at the center of the learning process. Digital devices become essential tools in the hands of students, opening the door to a more interactive, engaging and personalized educational experience. This leads to an evolution in the role of teachers, who become guides and facilitators of learning rather than mere dispensers of knowledge.

In this context, students take a more active role in their learning, exploring topics of interest to them through online resources and collaborating with peers from around the world. Global connectivity offers unprecedented learning opportunities, giving students access to a wide range of knowledge and cultural perspectives.

However, with the abundance of information available online, new challenges also arise. Students must learn to critically evaluate sources and discern between reliable information and misinformation. In addition, overuse of technology can lead to problems related to screen addiction and mental health.

It is therefore essential that digital education be balanced and inclusive, ensuring that all students have equitable access to digital resources and are able to develop the skills needed to navigate the evolving digital world. This means teaching them not only how to use technology, but also how to do so responsibly, critically and ethically.

In conclusion, the future of digital education offers significant promise, but also complex challenges to be faced. With a holistic, student-centered approach, we can prepare future generations to succeed in an increasingly digital world, enabling them to seize opportunities and navigate challenges with confidence and awareness.

I hope this book has given you the right keys to understanding how to approach technology and how to raise the new generation to it. It is a very important goal in everyone's life not to risk being overwhelmed by it. Technology is evolving much faster than we are able to assimilate. Knowing how to use it in our favor is a great help in our everyday lives; keeping it at bay is the big difference between using it consciously and being totally addicted to it! Our sanity and safety can be jeopardized by all this bombardment of media and information. It is a real new world, with its own rules and risks. Let us navigate it with awareness.

 I thank you for reading "Smart Generation: Technology, Education, and the Well-Being of Youth" and wish you an enjoyable journey into the Web and its possibilities!

www.ingramcontent.com/pod-product-compliance
Lightning Source LLC
Chambersburg PA
CBHW050822250726
48653CB00006B/2380